ROAD WARRIOR PHYSICIAN

Locum Tenens a How-to Guide

Elizabeth Noel Lumpkin

Dedication

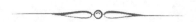

While the bulk of this book is based on my own experience, I've had the benefit of sharing the challenges and triumphs of similarly situated colleagues. In particular, I would like to note Ashok Shroff, Cheryl White, Larry Becker, Val Carrier, and especially, Bob Rockwell. These fellow anesthesiologists have all worked with me in various locations doing locums work. While they are temporary workers–itinerant laborers, you could say–their dedication is deep and constant. Each has shown me by example the value of giving your best effort regardless of the quality of the assignment. We have shared laughs and frustrations. I have learned something of value from each one of them. It is to these fine friends, my fellow travelers of whom I am so fond, that I dedicate this book.

Acknowledgement

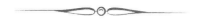

It is my belief that anyone who says that they wrote a book all by themselves is a liar or a fool–or both. While the work of writing is primarily a solitary occupation, it takes the support of many more individuals to create a book.

First, I would like to thank the people at Self-Publishing School (SPS) who created a system for encouraging others to write and publish their works. Can you write a book in a matter of weeks and get it published? Yes, you can! Having others who share your journey make it all the more agreeable and achievable.

My coaches, Hahna Kane Latonick and Ramy Habeeb, provided thoughtful insights. Both of these best-selling authors shared remarkable advice based on their professional experience, and I am confident that I would not have made it this far without their encouragement.

To my "acountabilibuddy" Marta Goertzen who shared weekly with me about the ups and downs she experienced and listened patiently to my rants, I am grateful for the meaningful conversation and for the gift of her friendship. I look forward to being a published author with you!

It is said that in cooking, three elements are important: taste, texture and presentation. While I thought that my book had taste, it was through the help of my editor Francine Rudd that the texture was improved and the presentation was enhanced. I learned so much in this process. I cannot thank her enough for her patience and sense of humor.

Finally, I thank my gracious family who has been there all along–before, during and after this entire project, and who have reminded me more than once, we are all a team.

About the Author

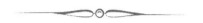

Elizabeth Noel Lumpkin is an anesthesiologist who has been doing locum tenens work for over a decade. Her career has taken her all over the United States and overseas on several medical missions. Graduating from Salem College, she worked for several years before returning to medical school at the University of Missouri-Columbia. She completed her residency at the Mayo Clinic in Rochester, Minnesota and a fellowship at Virginia Mason Hospital in Seattle, Washington.

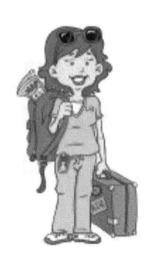

Outside of medicine, she enjoys travel (go figure!), reading, hiking, cooking and is a huge Jeopardy! fan as well as an avid solver of the New York Times crossword puzzle (see <u>lovethecrossword.com</u> for her blog devoted to this topic). It has long been a dream to create a book for others who are curious about this type of medical practice. Look for updates on this book and the locums lifestyle on her website <u>doctorlumpkin.com</u>.

After living all over the United States, she now calls the state of Washington her home. She lives there with her mother, two dogs, several koi and one eccentric parakeet.

A Cordial Invitation

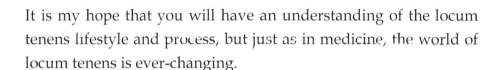

It is my hope that you will have an understanding of the locum tenens lifestyle and process, but just as in medicine, the world of locum tenens is ever-changing.

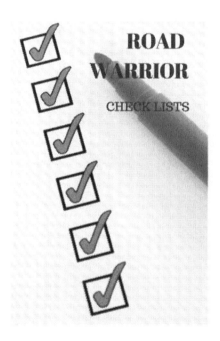

With that in mind, my website doctorlumpkin.com will feature updates on the current activities and trends of locum tenens. It will also showcase products, apps, and sites that can make your locums experience easier, perhaps less stressful and more rewarding.

I welcome your comments, suggestions and any stories you have to share.

To tempt you to make your first visit to the website, I've uploaded the <u>checklists</u> that you'll find in Chapter 6. Look for this logo!

Table of Contents

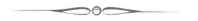

CHAPTER 1

About Locum Tenens

They've asked me to do this temporarily. I don't know what that means. Life is temporary.

Bob Schieffer

In this chapter, we'll discuss: How did this locums thing start? How long has it been around? Is there a role for locums in the future?

Definition and History

Locum Tenens is described in Merriam-Webster.com: [lō'kəm ten'ənz] Etymology: L, locus, place, tenere, to hold–a physician who is contracted to work on a temporary basis to fill in for a vacancy, vacation, or extended leave.

While there is some discussion about how locum tenens began, most agree that the concept emerged at the University of Utah in the 1970s. Given credit most often are Therus Kolff, MD, MPH and Alan Kronhaus, MD. They were working at the university on a project called Health Sciences Research Institute (HSRI) in conjunction with the Robert Wood Johnson Foundation. The foundation gave a grant to HSRI to study how to recruit physicians to work in the rural and underserved areas in the state.

The results of their study showed that physicians who were willing to work in the rural communities would do so if there was a method in place that would allow for occasional time off. The success of this program was evident, and soon Kronhaus was given permission by HSRI to start his own stand-alone locum tenens service. Within one year, they had expanded beyond the state and into other specialties.

Locum Tenens Today

Today, there are over 25 companies dealing exclusively with locum tenens physicians in all specialties, the industry generating $2 billion plus annually. From its early beginnings as a pilot study in 1970 to the formation of the first locum tenens agency in 1979, the industry has continued to play an increasingly large role in the healthcare field.

Clearly this is not a new trend, and it certainly is not going away.

From its inception, the face and practice of locum tenens has undergone a sea change. Prior to 2009, the average locum tenens physician was a new graduate who was testing the waters before committing to a full-time position. Groups who hired them did so primarily to cover vacations of their roster of providers.

Today, however, over 70% of locums providers have over two decades of experience. Coverage for vacations is now number three on the list of reasons that organizations need coverage. Today the number one reason by far is to fill a vacancy of a provider who has left the practice.

Many administrators were astonished to learn that in 2014, 90% of organizations employed a locum provider at some point–an astonishing 22% increase over the previous year!

Growing Trends

The statistics are alarming–but it should come as no surprise as there is a nationwide physician shortage. Most are unaware, however, of how large it already is and how much it will continue to grow in the coming decade.

In my specialty, anesthesiology, our own American Society of Anesthesiology looked at the 2002 numbers, which already indicated a shortage. They then predicted a shortage of 4,500 anesthesiologists by the year 2020.

For primary care, the outlook is even bleaker. In 2012, there was a shortage of 9,000 providers, and in 2020, the shortage is predicted to grow to over 65,000.

Survey Said. . .

Given these numbers, assume some of these issues will be on the horizon. There will be longer waits to see a physician and trouble even getting a primary care provider. As physicians become overburdened, expect to see increasing dissatisfaction on both sides of the stethoscope from patients and providers.

Look to the future, because that's where you'll spend the rest of your life.

George Burns

The Future

With the numbers in hand, how does the future look for locum tenens? At a recent gathering for a Healthcare Staffing Summit, it was predicted that healthcare staffing revenue would reach $10.9 billion, an increase over 2014 by 7%. One of the strongest growth areas was locum tenens, which saw an increase in revenue of 8% in 2014 with an anticipated 8% again in 2015.

Today with the face of healthcare changing and more physicians becoming employees, it has added a new dynamic to the practice of medicine–turnover. In the past, self-employed physicians had a great incentive to put down roots in the communities where they practiced, but no longer. As a result, hospitals are now seeing a greater number of physicians leaving their facilities and seeking other opportunities. Couple this with the growing shortage of physicians and no way to replace them quickly, and the need for locum tenens is only going to rise.

Currently, managers expect to increase their staff physicians by 31%, according to a Medical Economics article, as well as 7% expecting to increase the number of temporary physicians they use in the coming year. At present, primary care physicians are the most requested and are likely to continue to be in the future as their specialty is expecting the biggest shortage. In 2002, there were only 20,000 physicians working in a temporary capacity, the latest number is closer to 40,000 with primary care making up 17% of that total.

Other numbers that may surprise you, in 2002, there were 26,000 physicians who had done a locum tenens assignment; by 2014, that number surpassed 40,000. Far from being a way to make some extra money on occasion, locum tenens is fast becoming a line budget item for many healthcare facilities.

In 2012, the Department of Defense awarded over $50 million in contracts to finance locum tenens physicians through 2017. In 2015, the Veterans Administration used locum tenens providers in nearly all of their 1,400 facilities. At the same time, the Indian Health Service expanded healthcare coverage to the nearly 2 million Native Americans in their 160 facilities. In both of these cases, locum tenens were an essential part of the coverage. By now, you should understand that despite its modest beginnings, locum tenens has continued to develop and will certainly flourish in the future.

In the next chapter, we cover The Who–no, not that group–the people who do locum tenens, the motivations particular to each group as well as those incentives that overlap more than one group.

Resources

"Brief History of Locum Tenens - Icon." *Icon*. N.p., 21 Oct. 2015. Web. 14 June 2016.

Fellows, Jacqueline. "Use of Locum Tenens Up 22% in One Year." *HealthLeaders Media*. N.p., 13 Mar. 2014.

"Paging All Doctors! Combating the Physician Shortage (Infographic)." *Locum Tenens Daily*. N.p., 25 Sept. 2015.

Zimlich, Rachael. "The Rise of Locum Tenens among Primary Care Physicians." *Medical Economics*. Medical Economics, 8 Apr. 2014.

CHAPTER 2

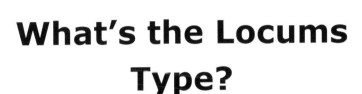

What's the Locums Type?

Be yourself; everyone else is already taken.

Oscar Wilde

Just who does locum tenens? I am glad you asked! Virtually every level of medicine and every specialty is represented. What are the advantages for the various groups and what are the motivations? Read on!

A number of years ago, when attending a meeting, I struck up a conversation with the woman sitting next to me, who happened to also be an anesthesiologist. We talked for a while, and the subject of where we each worked came up. She told me that she worked for six months of the year in an academic practice teaching residents critical care, and the remainder of her time she working doing locum tenens.

I was puzzled by this because, in my group, we had used locum tenens for the occasional coverage needed when someone had surgery. In years past, they had also hired locums when they were in the midst of looking for a new member for the group. But someone who did locums on a regular basis–well, that was definitely something new to me!

As we talked further, I learned what motivated her to take this direction. The academic center where she worked could not offer her full-time employment at the time of her hiring, so she sought a way to make ends meet, assuming that she would go full-time when the opportunity presented itself. She began doing locum tenens at that time and found that she enjoyed the freedom it gave her as well as the flexibility to do different cases (or actually do cases unlike many of her academic colleagues).

To her own surprise, when she was offered a full-time teaching position, she politely turned them down because she found that this hybrid of practices suited her quite well. In fact, she really could not imagine doing things any differently.

So who does locum tenens? There are several groups of individuals, and just like medicine in general, there is no one type of person. There are four main groups found in this part of medicine:

- Newly graduated residents
- Retired or soon-to-be retired physicians
- Mid-career physicians
- Full-time locums providers

As you can see from the list, it pretty much covers everyone in medicine these days. So what are the motivations that are common to each?

Newly Graduated Residents

The idea that a new resident might choose to do locum tenens comes as a surprise to many as they think that the main focus of your last year of residency is finding the right job. Many of the lectures and brainstorming sessions were about finding a permanent job, not a temporary one. However, there are many reasons that a short-term job might be the best fit:

- Having a spouse who is still completing residency or fellowship
- Having a spouse who is in the military
- Checking out new areas before committing

Retired or Soon-to-Be Retired

While the idea of retirement is appealing to many, there are those who still desire to continue working, just not as much. Of course, your current group or practice may be eager to hire you as a locum–you are a known quantity after all! On the other hand, the desire to be nearer to children and grandchildren can also provide the impetus for looking for work somewhere else.

It is not unusual to see a physician who is retired from the military (often at an astonishingly young age) who still wants to work, but without the commitment required for a full-time job. It can be a great boon to a practice–having a seasoned physician who wants to work without getting on the partnership track.

Mid-career Physicians

Some are frankly puzzled by the idea of someone who is established in a practice doing locums for someone else. There are many who do so for several reasons. Depending on the local economy and the economy in general, some choose to supplement their income by doing locums especially when the workload is lighter or even during their vacation times. In fact, I had a partner who did locums taking his family to the various locations. They played during the day while he worked, and they all enjoyed the new area in the evenings and weekends.

Sadly these days, the dissatisfaction among physicians is at an all-time high, so many are considering a job change or even a career change. Working elsewhere can often illuminate the source of the problem. Maybe it's the current location or even the career itself.

Like the previous category, there are those who do retirement planning by working in a new area–taking the time to check out the area as well as laying the groundwork for some part-time work down the road if the need and desire arise.

The Full-Time Locums Physician

If I had a dollar for every time someone asked where my permanent job was, I could retire myself! Even some recruiting agencies are surprised to find someone who does this for a full-time job, and yet I see more and more people choosing this route.

Initially, a disruption in a group or practice may result in many being without full-time employment with locums being a lifesaver. Over time, some find the new way of working suits them better than they would have imagined. Of course, many continue to do locums until the right permanent job comes along.

Another trend I have seen is those who are transitioning out of medicine into a new career choosing to do locums as a bridge until the new venture takes shape. I knew of one physician who developed his own sports line of nutritional products and did locums as a side line.

Flexibility

The story at the beginning of this chapter illustrates one major motivation for those who do locums work: flexibility. Most people give this as the primary reason they do locums; some, in fact, give it as the only reason. You choose for whom you work, and to a certain extent, you choose when you want to work. You are not wedded to some administrative ideal or infrastructure, and you may come and go without fear of losing your position, because you don't have a position with that practice except for the dates detailed in your contract.

Freedom

The attraction of greater freedom looms large. Naturally, there can be more free time as there are fewer non-work commitments attached to the locums provider-principally, fewer meetings. Of course, depending on the assignment, you may have evenings and weekends free. That definitely gives you more time to explore your new area, which may be one of the prime movers that brought you there in the first place.

Always bear in mind that this freedom while on the road does not necessarily translate into freedom once you return home. "Just what do you do with your free time?" many will ask me, not realizing that I return home to mail that has to be processed and other home projects that have been in standby mode while I've been on the road.

Financial

For some, the financial pull of doing locums is most influential. In the past, I have done assignments with lots of overtime and calls which yielded pretty sizable paychecks. These days, the cash cows are becoming scarcer as hospitals and groups are minding the bottom line more carefully. Of course, if you really want to work, there will always be groups hungry for your presence that will pay you accordingly.

In summary, you will find nearly every age level and experience level working as a locum tenens provider at various points in their career. It can benefit virtually anyone who seeks to learn from this type of employment.

In the next chapter, we'll cover the common question, where do you find the jobs? Do I want to work with an agency, and if so, how do I find a good one?

CHAPTER 3

Finding a Locums Job, Use an Agency or Not?

You got to be careful if you don't know where you're going, because you might not get there.

Yogi Berra

One of the most common questions I get is about finding a locum tenens job. The second, do you use an agency? Well, yes and no. All this and more is in the following pages . . .

When considering locum tenens, one of the first considerations will be just where do you want to go? Many will think initially of some idyllic location where you can lounge on the beach sipping a drink with an umbrella in it. But wait! That is a vacation we are talking about, not work. Just because you would like to take a paid vacation, don't think that anyone will be willing to finance it. You are doing locums work for just that–work. Being able to enjoy the local culture and surroundings can be a bonus, but only that. I have heard from some hospitals who talk about previous locums who had no interest in doing the work and only asked when they could go sightseeing or deep-sea fishing.

Just as at the inception of locum tenens, rural and, to some extent, underserved areas remain in need of coverage. They may not be the garden spot of their state, but they still need coverage. Depending on your motivation for doing locums, it is worth your while to take a good look at those options. Maybe you have no desire to go to Podunk, but if you go there, you may find a community that is more welcoming and more flexible than you would otherwise imagine.

Of course being willing to go to a more remote area is one thing; getting there can be quite another challenge. In looking at these areas, be sure to note where the nearest airport is and determine how long it might take you to get there. All of this will factor in when figuring out your travel options: how late might you arrive, do you need to go a day earlier, and so on.

There are also many practices in large cities that find a need for locums. They are likely to be more specific about their needs and less willing to pay extra as they often have a larger pool of local physicians from which to draw. So if they need locums coverage, they try to keep it to a minimum. In my own experience, I have found them less willing to pay for housing or paying a less than ideal wage if they are covering housing.

However, if you live in a larger metropolitan area, take the time to contact the various hospitals and practices in your specialty about potential needs. More than once, I have been presented for a job only to find out that they had found a local candidate to fill the slot.

The majority of the jobs you will hear about will be short-term assignments, usually a week to a few weeks. A good deal of this depends on your own specialty. In the case of mine, anesthesiology, jobs are usually in the weeks column. However, if you are interested in a long-term assignment covering months or a year or more, two main options exist: the Indian Health Service and the Veterans Administration (VA).

Working for either the Indian Health or the VA comes with its own pluses and minuses. I have not personally worked for either, but I have spoken with those who have. The credentialing for the VA is through its own particular system called VetPro. It is the same form used for permanent hires, so expect a long lag time before actually going to work for them.

Online

When you first consider locums work, the search itself can seem daunting. Just where do you look? One of the first places to look online. Simply typing "locums positions" will yield a plethora of choices. With that in mind, it is often worthwhile to choose filters such as specialty, whether locums or permanent, and perhaps most importantly, what states you are considering. The list is not exhaustive, but it is rather extensive just the same. Of course, you may see multiple listings for the same job, making reading it a bit tedious. It is still a worthwhile jumping-off place. In any case, it should give you a rough idea of the demand for locums in your field.

Your own specialty will have a jobs board often with a temporary, PRN or locums category. Anesthesiology has a site called Gaswork.com which lists jobs for permanent, locums, PRN, part-time and even fellowships. The database can be sorted using all states or specific states, and there are international listings. The upside to using your own specialty's site is that the number of listings is shorter, and as a rule, the site is better maintained as compared to the internet in general.

Agencies

As mentioned, there are now over 25 locums agencies in the United States. Simply Googling the phrase "locum tenens" will bring up the sites of the largest ones. Again, the question becomes, just which one or ones do you choose? Certain criteria are important to your search:

➢ NALTO (National Association of Locum Tenens Organizations) is a voluntary membership site for organizations recruiting locums providers. They have stringent requirements that must be met and maintained to remain a member. Most who belong will state this on their website. If an agency does not belong, I would want to know why. Belonging is a measure of integrity and a matter of pride for an organization. I would not work for an agency that does not belong.

➤ Areas served: Most will tell you that they can place someone in any state, which is true. But a quick look at the jobs posted for your specialty will often reveal a geographic bias. There is nothing wrong with this; it usually reflects the location of the agency. If they are located in Pennsylvania, it makes sense that many of their jobs will be found in and around the Northeast. Of course, if you want to work in the West, it might be better to look at another agency that at least has some jobs listed near there.

➤ Location of the agency: Tied to the above reason is the location of the agency. I live on the West Coast, making it difficult to communicate with an agency on the East Coast. More than once, I have had a recruiter call me in the wee hours of the morning about a potential job, not realizing the time difference. It can be difficult to find an agency that is close to your home base, but always keep the time zone difference in mind when calling them and having them call you.

➤ How many agencies? When I first started doing locums, I had only signed with one agency (the one a colleague referred to me). I soon learned that you should be listed with at least two agencies–in many cases for all of the above reasons. Some agencies have contacts that others do not, and it is eye-opening to see how two agencies in the same field can operate very differently. If you are just starting, I suggest you use two agencies, and if another is strongly recommended, go with three. More than that and you will quickly find your email and voicemail inboxes inundated with solicitations for work.

Some will tell you that they never work with an agency; others will tell you that they only work with an agency. So what are the pluses and minuses of working with one?

Agency Pluses

➢ Numbers: First and foremost, you have a contact that has multiple contacts. They will often have established relationships with hospitals or practices. Those relationships can streamline the process for you.

In terms of numbers, there are also numbers of people who can assist you with the process of locating a position. First, there is the recruiter, who is the primary person you will be talking to as well as to the client. Ideally, they should be well-acquainted with the client and have answers to your many questions about the job.

Second, there are other individuals who will be assisting you with credentialing (<u>covered further in Chapter 4</u>). Credentialing in the past usually took a few weeks; now, however, it can take several months. Having another person keeping track of all of those details can be a real time-saver. Third, you will have a contact number in the event that things do not go as planned. I know because I was stranded at an airport on New Year's Eve and was able to call the agency person and get another flight and hotel on short notice.

➤ Licensing: Check with your agency about their ability to help with the licensing process. If you do enough locums, odds are that you will have to get at least one more and likely several more state licenses to work for a certain client. Just like credentialing, the licensing process is fraught with tedium. Having someone at your agency who understands the intricacies of a certain state's regulations can save you from many headaches.

➤ Malpractice Insurance: Though you may have your own malpractice insurance, if you are going to another state, it may not cover you. When I first started, there was not a lot of work in my state, so I looked elsewhere. I checked with my own malpractice carrier and found that they would cover me in my home state, but not any other state.

➤ Getting paid on time: Having worked both agency and non-agency jobs, I have found one of the biggest hurdles with a non-agency job is getting paid in a timely fashion. Most are quite amenable to setting up a schedule and agreeing to the terms well before starting. One incident I clearly recall required multiple phone calls and emails before I finally got paid weeks after finishing the job. That was when I learned the value of an agency which gives you the exact pay date as well as the details regarding that pay.

Agency Minuses

➤ They work for their client. Let's be clear here. Though they may call you incessantly and bombard you with emails to get you to take that job, their loyalty is to their client. Making the client happy is their first priority; making you happy is second. That does not mean that they won't work to make your job more appealing, but never forget you're in second place in their heart.

➢ They're the middleman. The client comes first with the agent because the agent works on commission, which is a cut of what their client pays. The difference between what the client pays them and what you receive can be substantial. Of course, the agency is taking care of the travel details, credentialing, licensing and malpractice. Naturally, the agents have costs to cover. And this is one of the main reasons many choose to go solo when doing locums, and perhaps more importantly, why many smaller hospitals and practices choose to deal directly with locums.

➢ There's wide variance in the level of professionalism from agency to agency. Talk to those who do locums. Each of us is likely to have a story about someone at an agency who was "out to lunch," a little less than detail oriented, or no help in clearing an inevitable hurdle. Some of the details will surface when you first talk to them (See Chapter 6 for the <u>Recruiter Checklist</u>). Others will come to light when you start working with them. Getting a good recruiter to work with you is a real plus; having an idiot is a real minus.

Working Solo

Working without an agency can seem like working without a net.

And sometimes you'll miss having agency backup. Many full-time locums, however, are more than content to eliminate the middleman. So besides being your own boss, what are the ups and downs of this way of going solo?

First, you are in control. That seems obvious enough. You decide on which jobs to pursue and when you want to work. You arrange all of your own travel. That way, things are done to your liking. Sounds good, and it is. As physicians, many of us are more than accustomed to making our own decisions, so this seems natural.

Second, the money comes to you without someone else taking a cut of it. Financial considerations are one of the biggest reasons to go it alone. The difference in money can be more than enough to compensate for taking care of all the details yourself.

So what makes doing non-agency work less than ideal? Well, taking care of all those details yourself can be rather tedious at times. Credentialing (See Chapter 4.) has become a byzantine path to getting privileges at hospitals, and the phone calls and faxes required before completion can eat up substantial amounts of your time. Then there's the licensing process which has a never-ending supply of annoyances to boost that blood pressure of yours.

Of course, there are some fortunate folks who have a spouse or partner take care of the majority of these details. If you are thus blessed, then count yourself lucky indeed. Frequent gifts are strongly recommended by this author!

In summary, where can you do locums? Almost anywhere. Do you use an agency or do you work independently? Yes and yes.

In the next chapter, we get down to the nitty gritty–how to prepare for the first assignment, your first day orientation and even what to pack. Fasten your seat belts!

CHAPTER 4

---∋○⊂---

Get Ready, Get Set, Show Up!

As for any other journey, good planning will make things go more smoothly in your locums travel. In this chapter we'll cover what to ask an agency and how to find out details about your assignment. We'll also pass on ideas about creating a plan for your first day, and that all-important credentialing process.

Etiquette

Good manners reflect something from inside–an innate sense of consideration for others and respect for self.

Emily Post

Some of you are wondering why I would include a section on etiquette. We should have all learned basic manners at home or in school, but sadly, there are those who need a refresher course. When you are a temporary employee, there are even more subtleties that are worth remembering. Some of these will seem basic; others might give you food for thought.

➢ Show up–Seriously? I've been to more than one hospital where the person in charge has said to me, "Oh, good! You showed up!" After staring at them for what seems like a full minute, they usually explain that, about a third of the time, the locums provider they hire does not bother to show up. They agreed to a job only to have a better offer show up days later. Of course, I would rather have the better assignment, but an agreement is just that. Honoring your word may be out of fashion, but it will pay dividends when you are the locum.

Blessed are the flexible, for they shall not be bent out of shape. Anonymous

➢ Be flexible–This can be a tough one. Maybe you have won a Nobel Prize for Medicine, perhaps you are editor of the *New England Journal of Medicine,* or maybe you've just done things a certain way and you cannot see any other way of doing them. Well, put those notions of supremacy behind you. Being flexible with your assigned tasks will put you ahead of others who refuse to do certain cases, patients, etc.

One place where I had worked several times hired an additional locums in my absence for some weeks that I could not cover.

"How did it work out?" I asked the head of anesthesia.

"Terrible," he told me.

While she had said that she did "all" cases, when she arrived, she was assigned to one of the neurosurgeons. "I don't do neuro," she said.

"Don't do neuro?" they asked. This was a place with not one, but three busy neurosurgeons. *What happened to "all" cases?*

They managed the work for the two weeks she was assigned. Needless to say, she was not asked back. This does not mean that you should take on cases for which you are not trained or you cannot do. But making yourself adaptable to any and all situations will be considered a bonus. Of course, honesty is a plus.

➢ Neatness counts. Leave only footprints; take only photos, or your mother doesn't work here–It works for camping, houseguests, and for locums as well. At your home base, perhaps you have a minion who follows you around and picks up after you. Lucky you! Even with that being the case, unless you are bringing your minion with you, please try not to leave obvious signs that you have been there. Like so much of this, it seems obvious, but trust me, it will be noticed if you leave a trail of debris wherever you go.

Getting Ready

Keep calm and fill out the next form.

Anonymous

You have decided to take the plunge and you are ready to make that phone call whether to a locums agency or hospital. There are certain items it will behoove you to have handy. Getting all these items prepared in advance will make the following steps in this process that much easier.

➢ School dates and diplomas–Fortunately, you only need from college forward, supplying the start and end dates of each school.

I actually had one place ask for a copy of my college diploma. When I sent it to the requester, they responded, "I can't read it!"

To which I replied, "That's because it's in Latin."

The thoughtful response? "Oh."

I was tempted to say, "You asked for it," but wisely, I think, did not.

Copies of all diplomas from college forward will, however, be required. Since getting copies of all those diplomas can be tricky, once you've got them corralled, save lots of frustration and time by making several copies of each, keeping one set in your personal file with the rest ready for mailing.

Treat all residencies, fellowships, etc. the same way with the start and end dates of all and copies of each credential.

While you're at it, it will be worth your while to keep a spreadsheet or at least a cover page with all the names of heads of programs and pertinent dates on the top of this list. You will need this information more times than I care to count.

➤ Certifications–ACLS, PALS, ATLS–You will need a copy of each as well as their expiration date. One thing to note about ACLS in particular, while there are many online courses available telling that they offer a card, not all places will accept those and will only accept AHA certified cards. Make sure you know this before you start any other work or you may find yourself scrambling to find a course in the days before you leave for an assignment.

➤ Board certification–Once again, a copy of that document with the dates is necessary. Also note if you have recertified. If you are not board certified, be prepared to tell when you will be taking the exam and all of the salient details.

➤ Work history–If you are just coming out of residency, this should be easy enough. For the rest of us, however, this can be a rather long and detailed list. Personally, I keep a spreadsheet in Excel for this information. One important detail–get the phone numbers and fax numbers of the person(s) who will be attesting to your work at their institution. This is usually human resources, but knowing this level of detail will definitely speed up the process. Merely looking up the hospital website and jotting down the phone numbers listed is decidedly not sufficient. Drill down and find the appropriate extension so that the person handling your credentialing doesn't have to go through that frustrating process. This is someone you'd rather not frustrate–what goes around, comes around and always at the worst time.

➢ Current curriculum vitae–If you have not done so already, now is the time to format your CV for all of those places you will be applying. There are standard forms in Microsoft Word, but I use a program that allows me to easily update my CV after each assignment (yes, I update after I finish each assignment).

➢ Photo–Nice try using that photo from your college graduation! These days, they want one that was taken within the last six months. With everyone taking selfies, this should not be a huge problem, but avoid those that are part of a group photo, and choose a neutral background if at all possible. You can also go to many of the places that offer passport photos because they will be formatted for the required size.

One thing to note about the ID photo–it is easy to simply print one out, affix it to the form and think you are done with it. But this photo will likely end up in the medical directory, or even worse, on your staff badge. Make a judicious choice you won't live to regret!

➢ Licenses, DEA–While this seems obvious on the surface, as you will need a license and DEA wherever you go, you will also need a photocopy and dates of any inactive license(s). As with the schools above, I recommend a master list with all of the dates (active and inactive) as this is information that you will need again and again.

➢ CME–You need it to renew your licenses, and now you will frequently need it for credentialing as well. There are several programs online and apps as well that can help you keep all of this information in a tidy form. I use <u>myCME Bank</u>.

➢ Case logs–If you kept a case log or some other type of log during residency, get ready to use it again! Certainly in my own specialty, case logs or at least percentages are now required for updating files, so compile some sort of document with the necessary details.

➢ References–Depending on the agency, hospital or practice, you will typically need anywhere from two to six references. It should go without saying that these should be in your own specialty, at least the majority of them should be. As with the schools and work history, get phone numbers with extensions if applicable, fax numbers (if they have them) and email addresses. I am usually leery of giving the personal addresses of any references, so a complete work address has always functioned for me.

Naturally, you should ask each individual if they are willing to provide a reference for you. It will usually entail a phone call or an emailed form. If you are currently working, your references should be people who have worked with you in the last two years.

Once you've gathered all of this information, you are ready to make that call. If they have questions right away about dates or license info, you'll have it right at your fingertips, and you'll look like a locums rock star! The above information will be needed to get credentialed with a locums agency, hospital, practice or new state license.

I used to carry hard copies of all of the above. Later on, I put it all on a flash drive. These days, I have everything in <u>Evernote</u>. I highly recommend it. The basic program is free (can't beat the cost!). It will make organizing your locums life that much easier.

Tools for the Road

You survived credentialing, and now you have to get your gear in gear! What do you take with you on your assignment? Besides the obvious, what are some of the things that will make your life easier on the road?

Why buy good luggage? You only use it when you travel.

Yogi Berra

➢ Luggage–Despite what Yogi Berra thought, having good quality luggage is going to serve you well. After going through several types of luggage, I found the lighter weight, hard-shell bag with wheels that rotate in all directions a very worthwhile investment. Buy two, one for carry-on and one for checking. You will be schlepping your bags through airports and hotels, on sidewalks, and in various types of ground transportation. Be good to your back; you only have.

➢ Kitchen supplies–No, I am not suggesting that you take your Mixmaster and food processor, but at a minimum take a mug, a set of flatware, and plate for eating on the road. While takeout places will offer plastic forks and knives, few give you plates. You may be a fan of eating out of those little sections in your Styrofoam container. I, for one, am not. I purchased a set of bamboo flatware (chopsticks included!) which I am able to carry with me, even on the plane. They are easily washed and have lasted for years. I also bought a plastic plate and cup which I pack in my bag.

➢ Laundry–If you are gone for more than a week, you will probably have to do laundry while on the road. Most hotels offer washers and dryers that typically cost $2.00 per wash and dry cycles. The hotels will also offer to sell you detergent and dryer sheets at an incredible cost. I have a small pack in which I keep rolls of quarters, Tide pods and dryer sheets. I also have a laundry bag that makes my life so much easier.

➢ Battery-operated alarm clock–Since every hotel has an alarm clock, why bring your own? My two-word answer is power outage. You might be thinking overkill, just how often does that happen? It only takes one power outage to make you appreciate having your own clock that laughs at fluctuations in the power grid. My travel clock has a nifty feature, an LED flashlight that's been useful in a number of situations.

First Day Jitters

I'm a stranger here myself.

Ogden Nash

More than anything else, people ask me, "How do you find your way around at a new place? I could never do that." We can all identify with the anxiety that comes from going to a new place for the first time, starting a new job, etc. As a full-time locums provider, it is something that I do on a routine basis. Are there tricks to make it easier? You bet there is!

Before leaving home

I like to do my initial reconnaissance before I ever start to travel. If you are going to be working at a hospital, they'll have a website, complete with photos, maps, etc. If you are going to work with a group, they'll probably have one too. Look up the department that hired you and note the names and photos that accompany. You don't have to commit these to memory (although it's a great mental exercise), but it will help on that first day when you are trying to connect with the person or persons that are anticipating your arrival.

If you've gotten your assignment through an agency, they will send you an itinerary and maybe even maps to get from the airport to the hotel and subsequently to the hospital. If they don't or if you've opted to get your position on your own, Google Maps or any of the online map apps should be able to fill in the blanks for you. Review the routes you will need to take. Often I get in late at night, and having some familiarity with the street and place names makes navigation a little less tedious.

Even if you don't think this is going to be a routine for you, it will serve you well to join loyalty programs of the airline(s) and hotel(s) you'll be using. Online check-in for airlines has been around for a while, and it saves you time and frustration when you arrive at the airport. Use your smartphone for your boarding pass. These days many airlines allow you to print your own baggage tags.

I check in online for my hotel as well. This cuts the time spent at reception. Usually giving your name will result in your room cards being handed to you without any further ado.

Perhaps most important, have copies of all the necessary documents, especially your state license and DEA, either as hard copies, scans on your phone or flash drive. More than once, I have needed proof. Despite having passed the required credentialing, the hospital was unable to locate my license. Thankfully, I had a copy with me. Human resources is not usually open for business when I start my day, so having this on hand prevented yet another delay.

While on the road

There are few things that are more frustrating than to be delayed while en route to your assignment. It happens, so be prepared for it. Keep all travel emergency contact numbers handy. This is one of my prime Evernote uses. Note any additional flights in and around yours in case of delay or cancelation. Have the main phone number of the hospital or practice. Your delay may come after hours, but you can always leave a message in the event you won't be showing up at the appointed time.

If you arrive early enough, take a test drive to the hospital or office the night before just to develop a little comfort with the route. When doing this, you can usually find where to park at least on that first day. Many hospitals will use your ID badge for parking; some require you to get a separate tag. Almost all will allow you to use visitor parking for the first day. All of this will save you time and anxiety on that first morning.

First day

Learn your lines and don't bump into the furniture.

Noel Coward

Your first day will give you a glimpse into the general milieu of your hospital. Orientation on that day varies greatly. Perhaps no other feature has such a range as the way hospitals or groups orient you. To illustrate this, I offer two extreme examples.

Hospital 1

I arrive, prepared with everything to start my first day. "Who are you?" the person at the OR desk asked.

"I am your locums anesthesiologist," I reply politely.

"Another one?" she queries suspiciously.

"I am looking for the anesthesiologist in charge today, if possible."

"Who's in charge today for anesthesia?" she barks to those around.

Puzzled faces stare back at me. "Can I at least go to the locker room and change?" I ask.

Fingers point in the general direction of the locker room. Once in the locker room, I find my scrubs and am changing when another physician walks in. As luck would have it, she is one of the other locums anesthesiologists. We introduce ourselves and she fills me in on the details about the practice there.

When we arrive at the OR desk, I am informed which OR I will be covering with no further information given. When I get to my room, I learn that I am doing a thoracotomy, a rather involved case, especially for someone who is still trying to figure out where everything is. Next I learn that the anesthesia tech that always helps with this is on vacation. None of the permanent staff step up to help me get started, but the other locums does.

Hospital 2

Prior to my arrival, I get an email from one of the permanent staff, introducing himself and giving me details about the hospital and the usual cases covered. When I arrive at the hospital, I am greeted by name by the charge nurse. Then the anesthesiologist in charge that day gives me a sheet with all of the phone numbers and access codes that I will need to get around the hospital. He then accompanies me to the pharmacy to make sure that my Pyxis access is in order and then introduces me to the rest of the staff.

I am given details and information about my first case and my surgeon. The anesthesia tech assists me with my first case to make sure I know where everything is. Later on in the day, when he is busy with another room, the anesthesiologist in charge checks on me to make sure that I have everything I need. Later that week, he and his wife have me over to their house for dinner to find out how things are going.

While these two examples are extreme, they illustrate how much preparedness counts when you encounter Hospital 1. Chances are, that even there, you can find an ally who is willing to assist you, some empathetic soul who already knows the drill and is willing to share it with you.

Back in the day when I first started doing locums, I would carry a blank sheet of paper and on it write names and various bits of information that I would need. I would even write descriptions of people to help me remember their names! Of course, I would also draw maps, codes I would need to remember, etc.

Say cheese!

I now use my phone camera to take pictures of people (after asking, of course) and send them to <u>Evernote</u> where I store all salient information needed for my assignment. This becomes invaluable if you return to a facility and helps avoid those embarrassing "I'm sorry, but I cannot recall your name" moments; in fact, you'll look like the megastar you are when you can recall someone's name and how they helped you previously.

Your cell phone camera can also capture snapshots of forms that you may need for orders, etc. Much of this has been replaced by the electronic medical record (EMR), but I never fail to be amazed by how much paperwork still exists in today's hospitals.

All those tags and badges

At the very least, take a Ziploc bag with you to contain all of the tags, badges, etc. Your own bag can quickly become swamped with papers and items that you will acquire on your first day. I started using one of those zipper pouches that are in the school supply section of many stores.

It is useful because the mesh will allow you to see what badges you have, and the zipper will hold any pertinent items you want to keep safer, like a locker key or a pager. This is also useful for any return trips to the facility because I keep all of the items in their own folder at home. When I am heading out, I just put the folder in my bag, and I am ready to go!

Paperwork again!

As I stated previously, there seems to be no end to paper use. You will most likely need a time sheet. If you are working with an agency, they will usually email you this with all of your travel information, etc., but be ready with your own. If you are working for a group directly, they may have a form to give you on the first day. It is your responsibility to fill it out and submit it in a timely fashion. Many agencies are very particular about this, so it is prudent to make note of their deadline for receiving this.

Make sure you know the name and the fax number of who will be processing your time sheet. On the first day, make a point of finding out who is responsible for signing it and if you can fax it directly from the hospital, as many will want a copy of your time sheet before you leave. I always keep a copy (scanned into Evernote, naturally!) in the event that someone tries to tell me that they did not receive it.

Always looking to the future, you should get names and phone numbers with extensions of individuals willing to be a reference for you at a later date. Most are perfectly agreeable to do so while some for whatever reason are reluctant to provide references, but you should be able to find a couple of people who can vouch for you later on. These should also be entered in Evernote or whatever database or folder you choose.

Meanwhile, back at the ranch . . .

You have survived your first day, perhaps the first week, and now that you have taken a moment to relax, you are faced with the prospect of four hotel walls staring back at you. I'll admit that initially the idea that someone is making your bed every day and cleaning your bathroom sounds pretty good, great even. However, after a couple of weeks, the sparkle starts to dull and by the third week, much less the fourth, you feel yourself going a little crazy. How do you survive living on the road and out of a suitcase?

Food, glorious food!

Eating out is the obvious answer when you first arrive in a new place, but this can wreak havoc on your wallet as well as your waistline. While I enjoy trying new restaurants, I prefer to have more control over what I eat. It saves me money on food and the inevitable new wardrobe.

In almost every place you go, there is a grocery store, so take a trip there and buy some supplies for your stay. Assuming you have a small refrigerator in your room, I recommend buying breakfast items in particular. I often stay in a hotel that offers breakfast, which usually starts around 6:30 when I must be leaving for the hospital, so I try to have breakfast in my room.

I often have yogurt and some oatmeal from the microwave that almost every hotel room has. As I mentioned previously, I travel with a set of utensils, a small collapsible bowl, a plate, and a cup. That way, I can have oatmeal or soup and make a variety of dishes that can be eaten without digging into a container. There is something more dignified about eating off of a plate rather than Styrofoam. Call me old-fashioned, but that's the way I am!

If your job is similar to mine, lunch is often like a unicorn, a fantasy you hear about but never see. Taking something with you to work is going to save you on those long days. I like to carry trail bars, dried fruit and nuts. They take up a minimum of space, require no heating or cooling, and can be eaten quickly between cases or patients.

Dinner can be the tricky one as your hotel room may not offer a great selection of appliances. If you want to avoid eating out, what can you do? Of course, there are microwaveable selections available, some of them quite good, but again, you can eat more calories than you want if you go this route too often.

Those rotisserie chickens that you see in almost every grocery store now make sense. They're ready to eat, and will last more than a couple of meals (at least for me). I buy some frozen vegetables and microwave them, and you have a complete meal for a fraction of the cost. The leftovers will work well for lunch (assuming you get time for lunch).

Staying fit

Supposing you are keeping your calorie intake in check, there is still the matter of staying reasonably fit. Maybe you are in top shape, participating in Ironman triathlons all over the map, but if you are like most of us, you will need some way to maintain your fitness while traveling. The hurdles are there: limited time, limited access to gyms, disruption of your routine, etc. You get the idea.

If you have a gym at home, whether in your town or your house, you obviously cannot take such things with you on the road. However, if you belong to a gym, ask if the local gym will honor your membership. Tell them your situation and many will be happy to accept you as a temporary member, sometimes for a small fee, sometimes for free!

If there is not a gym handy, check to see if your hotel has one. Though often vacant throughout the day, in the early morning hours they are frequently packed. Ask the reception desk about gym options as well. They sometimes have vouchers for the local gyms.

Personally, I prefer walking, the old-fashioned method of exercising. If possible, and daylight permitting, I will often walk to work. Yes, it takes a little more time, but by the end of the day, when I return to the hotel, my exercise is finished, and I can focus on other fun things instead! Walking is free, and many places now have trails marked throughout the area, so you can see a lot of the new town and get exercise to boot.

Getting out

The world is a book. Those who do not travel read only a page.

St. Augustine

You have the routine at work; things are going well. You're eating decently and getting some exercise, but if you really want to get a feel for all that there is, you need to leave the hospital and the hotel and get out. I was doing locums in Alaska when I talked to another locums there. After spending a weekend hiking in the local mountains and seeing all kinds of wildlife, I asked her what she did over the weekend.

"I read," she said.

"You read???" I asked, "Were you sick or something?"

"No," she said, "I like to read on the weekend."

"Don't you want to get out and see the local area? You're in Alaska, for goodness sake!"

"Nah, it doesn't really interest me."

Personally, I find such an attitude perplexing. Many of us state travel as a motivation for doing locums, and I can read almost anywhere, but I can't always go hiking in beautiful mountains and experience local culture, especially somewhere like Alaska.

So where do you go? Ask your fellow staff members, ask the hotel personnel, and above all, ask your patients. I find them to be the greatest sources of information about a local area. Through them, I have found amazing restaurants, great hikes, interesting museums, fantastic local scenery and the most entertaining golf course ever! The public library is also a great source of local events, many activities costing very little or maybe nothing at all.

As you can see, the details involved before you even start an assignment can be overwhelming. A little preparation early on will pay off down the road.

Credentialing Game Plan

This may seem like I am beating a dead horse, but credentialing is more than likely going to be the bane of your existence if you do locums, no matter what the length of the assignment. Back in the "old days," credentialing could take as little as two weeks, even a weekend in an emergent situation. Now, it takes months, sometimes several months. Unlike nurses, who can select an assignment and go there a week later, physicians have few similar options. So steel yourself for this process. It can get ugly; I promise you.

That being said, there are ways to organize things and hopefully diminish the pain. As I mentioned in Chapter 2, get all your documents together and get everything photocopied. Yes, that can mean taking your framed diplomas off the wall and bringing them to your local printing emporium. It sounds ridiculous, and it is, but you will probably need a copy of at least one of those diplomas at some point. Get the busy work out of the way early.

For the sake of argument, I will assume that you have all of the necessary documentation perhaps in a manila folder or in Evernote (my recommendation). If you have it all in a folder, do yourself a favor: Scan it into a computer, tablet, or some other device that you will have with you on the road. Scanner? Yes, a scanner. If you don't have one, get one, ideally one that is portable. Many tout the ScanSnap from Fujitsu; I have found the Doxie scanner to be even more portable, which is a real bonus for me. In any case, get a good scanner and use it.

Next you will need a fax. That's right, I said a fax. You may be thinking that they went out with the dodo, but change comes slowly to HR departments, especially in hospitals. You will probably be faxing weekly or even daily until this credentialing process is finished.

If you are like I am, you have a printer-fax-scanner combo and can fax things from home fairly easily. However, I do recommend considering an online fax service which will allow you to fax from anywhere at any time. If you have scanned everything into your computer, you can simply upload the necessary documents to your online fax, and voila! You are faxing with ease without the use of a landline.

Before you start faxing and scanning with abandon, get the names of all those folks who are going to be with you on this journey. Just who do I mean? The name of the person at your locums agency (assuming you are using one) and the person or persons in the human resources department who will be handling your file. Also, get the name of the department chair for which you will be working. Not just the names, get their phone numbers, fax numbers and cell phone numbers, if they offer them.

You will feel as though you are joined at the hip to some of these people by the time you arrive at their hospital. They will be calling and emailing you, so create a file for them along with your documents.

For the truly OCD (I count myself among them), keep a log of what you send and to whom you send the information. Then when person A tells you that they have not received document D, to which you reply, but I see that you received the fax on such and such a date. At the very least, it will give you smug self-satisfaction if nothing else. It will also tell them that you are on top of things. And in the best of cases, it will cause them to treat you accordingly.

Naturally, in spite of your best intentions, there will be items that you send and resend. Patience is a virtue that I continue to work on, especially in this situation. Getting angry at the person on the other end of the phone is not going to help and could potentially hurt you down the road. Resist the urge to tell them that their IQ is in single digits, no matter how much evidence you may have for your assessment.

When credentialing–and especially when applying for a new license–there are bound to be due dates for certain materials. Make a note of these and put them on your calendar. Use whatever system you have for reminders. If you don't have a system, get one. Despite the fact that there will be numerous individuals involved with your credentialing, you are ultimately responsible for getting all of the documentation in on time. I have heard of people who had assignments delayed for weeks or months or even canceled, all because of a credentialing glitch. Don't let this happen to you. Call, email or send smoke signals to those people above and make sure that they have everything they need.

One final note, if you continue to do locums work, your first go at credentialing will not be your last. Even at places where I have worked for years, I have to re-credential every two years just like the permanent staff. Being pleasant to folks that work with you on this will pay off, just like your mother told you! If someone is particularly helpful, I have been known to send flowers or some other gift thanking them. You may feel that you have arrived and that such actions are beneath you, but trust me, such actions do not go unnoticed.

Long-Term Locums

While this idea has been briefly covered in Chapter 1, it deserves additional mention. If you choose to make locums more than temporary, a means of making more money or finding a job, you will need to make certain adjustments in your lifestyle and how you organize it. The numbers of those who do choose to do this full time are small, but that should not dissuade you from considering it. Before doing so, allow me to offer some suggestions for making the transition easier.

➤ Travel apps, sites, etc.–It should come as no surprise that belonging to any airline reward program can be a benefit. Love it or hate it, you will probably be doing more than your fair share of air travel, so you might as well get some points for it. There are numerous sites out there that will cover the loyalty programs in detail, but my main suggestion for you is to choose the airline that you will be flying most often and look at its airline partners.

The quickest way to earn more points is by using all of the loyalty program partners. For example, I fly Alaska Airlines most often which partners with American and Delta (among others). When I fly either of those, I use my Alaska Airlines loyalty number when booking. Alaska divides the number of miles needed to attain elite status based on whether you flew on Alaska or its partners, but if you are traveling six months out of the year, you can attain elite status fairly quickly by using this method.

Hotels are another way of racking up the status points, and most agencies are more than happy to book you at a hotel in your chain of choice. Again, read the sites and see if you can get points on your airline program as well. To bring all of these sites together, I heartily recommend Tripit.com as an online source for amassing all of your travel information. When you get a confirmation email, all you have to do is forward it to Tripit, and they collate everything into a tidy itinerary for you. This is especially valuable if you are booking your own travel and want to remember that confirmation number or phone number when you are on the road.

➢ Paperwork–Despite the influx of EMR and the promise that "We would be paperless by 2010!" there seems to be no end the paperwork involved in medicine. While credentialing covers a good deal of this, as a long-term locums, you will be responsible for maintaining your CV as well as your CME records. In the past, you may have had a department that monitored the looming expiration of your state license or DEA, but now it's on your head to keep track of it. Most states as well as the DEA will send out notices to you well in advance, but keeping track of the CMEs you have earned (as well as the various requirements for each state) can be tedious.

For several years, I used the online site eeds.com. I entered the information each month and was able to produce a report at any time to cover whatever time period was necessary for a license or credentialing. All of this came at a price, but it was still a time saver, so I never complained.

Now, however, I am using MyCME.com, which offers a CME bank using an app on your iPhone or Android, and get this–it's free! So, the price is quite an incentive for using this site. I put a reminder in my Google calendar each month to update my CME. It is the best way I know to stay on top of this recordkeeping.

➢ Immunizations–By now, you have probably been presented with the requirement of getting an annual flu shot. In the past, it was probably offered to you while working at your hospital or office. Now, if you are not around when it is offered, it will be up to you to pay for it. That goes for PPD as well as tDAP, if they ask for it. If you use an outside source, get a copy of the record, snap a photo of it with your phone or tablet and keep it with you in whatever database you have (I prefer Evernote).

➢ ACLS, PALS, etc.–Ah, yes, those pesky certifications and courses that you need for almost every hospital and/or office. If you are like I am, those two years between certifications seem to vanish like the wind. Keep track of all expiration dates and bear in mind that you may not be able to take advantage of any course while you are working, so you will probably have to take an online course and schedule your skills session with a local provider. This can be painful, but in looking at the AHA site, you should be able to find someone in your area who can schedule a skills session for you.

Just make sure that you start looking early enough. There is nothing worse than having to scramble to find someone just to check you off on your ACLS the day before you leave for an assignment. Also, there are some hospitals that will only accept an AHA-certified card which requires you to be present for your skills session. There are several online ACLS re-certs which do not require your physical presence. But to be safe, it is probably wisest to go the conservative route and use the AHA courses. Doing so will eliminate the less than pleasant surprise of having to take the course again (at your expense, I might add).

➢ Life outside work–Your life at home is probably full of activities, but working on the road for six months of the year is going to drain you if you don't find pleasant diversions in the area you are working. I do not mean that you have to be going out every night, but I do suggest that you take the time to take a class or participate in some activity outside of work.

I have belonged to BSF (Bible Study Fellowship) and Toastmasters, both of which have chapters all over the United States (and the world for that matter). I look up the chapters when I am traveling and try to make it to the local meetings. Doing this has allowed me the opportunity to interact with people outside of medicine and forge new friendships.

In the next section, we turn the tables. We'll address those that do the hiring. What do you ask your prospects and how do you prepare? Get out the welcome mat!

CHAPTER 5

<hr/>

Hiring a Locums–the Other Side of the Coin

So let's be honest with ourselves and not take ourselves too serious, and never condemn the other fellow for doing what we are doing every day, only in a different way.

Will Rogers

When it is time for YOU to hire a locums provider, who do you call, what do you ask, and how do you prepare? They may be working for you, but a few actions on your part can make life easier for both of you.

If you work in the medical field long enough, odds are you will be considering hiring a locum tenens provider at some point. While the majority of this book is devoted to the locums lifestyle, I thought it would be helpful to point out things to consider when you are doing the hiring.

Be Specific

Nothing is more annoying than reading through a description of a facility needing locums coverage than to read, "Quality facility with beautiful community, perfect for the lover of the outdoors!" Seriously? Reading descriptions like these is like reading a real estate ad. Be wary of descriptions containing the words: charming, quintessential and paradise. If you need help with coverage, something is missing. It doesn't mean that your hospital isn't great, but it tells a prospective physician next to nothing about your practice or hospital.

I have had recruiters tell me grossly inaccurate information, not that they were lying intentionally, but because they had not received the right information. Sit down and think about what you really need for your coverage such as:

How long do you anticipate needing the coverage? I understand that you are watching your budget, but realistically, what is the coverage covering? If it is simply a vacation, then you probably are talking about a week or two.

However, if you are looking to hire an additional physician or a replacement, the process takes an average of eighteen months. During that time, you will want to be able to function effectively and introduce prospective hires to a staff that does not look overly stressed. Hiring a locums to help out can make this process much smoother. If you think that this is your situation, say so! Not everyone is looking for a short-term assignment. So if you have potentially ongoing needs, do not be hesitant to let the agency or provider know this.

Just what do you need coverage for? This covers what the actual duties will be. I am an anesthesiologist and certainly know what an anesthesiologist does, but what does the job require? Do they do neuro, spines or also heads? Cardiac? OB? Pediatrics? Those are just a few of the areas that should be delineated, but also, is there call? Is it in-house or pager? How frequent is it? If you want to be a real friend, describe what a typical night of call is like. Is it infrequent or are they up most of the night? Do they work post call? If there is no call, what will the average day look like?

Be Prepared

I find it intriguing that a group or hospital may be looking to hire someone and will go to great lengths to prepare for an upcoming interview, but when it comes to having a locums come to their practice, they do next to nothing to help them get oriented. Does it not occur to them that the locums might be looking to change jobs or at the very least, know those who are?

With all that in mind, it is my humble opinion that it just might make things work more smoothly if you prepare for a locums in the same manner as you would a potential addition to your staff.

Form a "your first day" checklist. It all depends on the hospital or office, but there are bound to be those ubiquitous little access codes these days. Get a list of those and give them out along with any other names, phone numbers, etc. that might come in handy.

Give a tour of your facility. While it might seem shocking to some, I have arrived at a hospital and after telling them of my status, have been told, "Oh, you're in OR 4." And that would be where, exactly? Fingers point in the general direction. While this example is extreme, it is more of the norm than you might imagine.

If at all possible, block out the first morning to give your locums a chance to get access at the pharmacy, get a badge and get a sense of the layout. This is especially true if he/she will be taking call. Have I ever arrived at a new place and been told I was on call the first night? You betcha. Don't do this. If you have any hope of hiring new staff, you have just eliminated one good source of leads by pulling this preposterously stupid stunt.

Let them know about your community. While they are not there to be entertained, give out some information about your corner of the world. What are the good restaurants? Are there any sites they should try to visit? Think about what you try to impart to those who interview. Even if they are not looking for a job, if you foresee long-term needs, letting them know more about the area will improve their chances of returning to your site.

Be Curious

Perhaps your group or hospital has all the answers. Maybe you never have a problem hiring new staff, and those who join never want to leave, everyone's spouse loves the community, and your administration never interferes with your job and only compliments your fine performance. If that's the case, package some of that pixie dust and start selling it on the open market, because you're one in a million!

Now, for the rest of you, at least one of those items above is not true, and it plays a role in why you need to hire a locums. If you have a locums working with you that you enjoy and respect, take the time to ask their honest opinion of your place. They might be hesitant to be too frank, but tell them if there's anything you would like to change and see what they might offer in response.

It's easy to think that your own facility is unique, and that all the problems you have are so different from other places, but in many cases, this is not true. Some of us have seen hospitals of all sizes in all areas of the country. While we've seen some real disasters, we've also experienced a few great places. Odds are we might have an idea or two that would help you.

While you're at it, if you truly like working with your current locums, why not share a meal with them? You might find that doing so will offer new insights into your practice and your community, not in a find-out-the-dirt way but more in the positive aspect of what you have to offer. I have found that when hospitals or groups are mired in the process of finding someone, they lose some of the enthusiasm they need to present to potential partners. So while it is beneficial to know the not so nice things, it is also good to know some of the pluses.

As I've mentioned, you do not have to entertain your locums, but in the interest of establishing a long-term relationship, think about including them in activities outside of the hospital. That long-term relationship can extend to not only returning to work at your facility but also referring other quality individuals to you or conversely, steering less than stellar ones away from you.

Be Polite

It may seem as though I am hammering the etiquette, but I cannot overstate what should be obvious: be polite to others, and they will usually return the favor. I have stated extreme examples of rudeness in this book, but there are less extreme ones as well. So let's cover just a few basics, shall we?

Ask them how things are going. Can this be any easier? If you take a vested interest in keeping things running smoothly, asking this question can open the channels of communication.

Offer help when necessary. Some of us are used to doing things on our own, but an offer of help is never a bad thing.

When possible, make sure that they get a breather during the day. We've all survived long hours without as much as a bathroom break. But if everyone else is getting a pause that refreshes, include your locums in the mix.

If you know that they will have to work with a difficult surgeon or patient, try and give them some warning and advice. Being thrown to the wolves helps no one and is potentially harmful to many.

Questions to Ask Your Prospective Locums

Your own hospital and the agency (if you used one) will have credentialed your applicant. But let's be honest, their questions often have nothing to do with the day-to-day practical issues that you are facing. I am never offended if a client wishes to talk with me prior to my arrival or even prior to starting credentialing; doing so can often clear up issues and questions well in advance. These are some of the questions that I have been asked in the past or perhaps some I wish that someone had asked!

➤ *Where are you currently working?* This is rather obvious, but asking more about the current practice will elicit what cases or patients they see most often. A quick search will tell you the size of the hospital and its general volume.

➤ *Why are you doing locums?* Some are doing it just to check out the market. Others are doing it to supplement their current income. Others like me do it full time. Certainly the motivations for each of these categories will be different. Those who are checking out the scene will be curious to know more about your practice overall as well as the community. If you are recruiting, this is definitely a prospective candidate until proven otherwise. Those wishing to supplement their income might be interested in overtime, call, etc. Ask! Naturally, anyone who tells you that they are in the market for a permanent job deserves a closer look.

➤ *What kind of cases do you see most often?* While I have been doing nearly every type of case since residency, certain assignments do not have them or limit them to permanent staff. When it comes to staffing rooms, this should alleviate some of the unpleasant surprises like finding out that someone has not done neuro cases since the Reagan administration!

> *What do you do in your free time?* Now, this is not necessarily any of your business, but as I've mentioned previously, knowing something more about the person outside of where they went to medical school and where they did residency, can add to your assessment. Plus, if you enjoy this person, knowing what they might like to do outside of work can offer you an opportunity to get to know them better, perhaps leading to a chance to recruit them or find out the name of someone who wants to be recruited.

> *How many locums assignments have you done?* This should be found on their CV, but ask anyway. If it is their first assignment, it is well worth knowing this ahead of time. Doing a locums assignment for the first time can be somewhat overwhelming for both parties. If this is the case, then consider assigning a mentor for at least the first day, if possible. Both of you will be grateful in the long run. If they have been doing locums frequently or for a long time, ferret out any pertinent positives and negatives about their experiences.

Of course, there will be questions that are tailored to your area and/or hospital. Asking the candidate about their knowledge of weather, culture, and the like will help them avoid certain problems. I recall one physician from southern Georgia who was unprepared for winter weather to appear in Alaska in early

October. Remember we don't all experience climates the same way!

In summary, taking the time to actually know your locums provider can lead to a mutually beneficial relationship. Even when you think it is going to be a short-term need, it never hurts to plan for contingencies. To paraphrase Mark Twain - Always be kind. This will gratify some people and astonish the rest.

CHAPTER 6

Making Lists & Checking Them at Least Twice

The human animal differs from the lesser primates
in his passion for lists.

H. Allen Smith

Calling your Recruiter Checklist–Questions to Have Ready

Agency information:

- name of agency
- name of recruiter

- phone number
- fax number
- cell number
- email address

Areas the agency covers:

- geographic
- medical specialties
- physicians only or all healthcare professionals

How long:

- Has the recruiter worked as a recruiter?
- Has the recruiter been with the current agency?
- Have they dealt with your current specialty?

How many:

- Clients do they manage?
- Providers do they manage?

Is there help with:

- Licensing
- Credentialing
- Travel

Malpractice coverage:

- Is with what company?
- How long have they used their current company?

- What are the limits?

Regarding the proposed assignment under discussion:

- Is it a new or old client?
- If it's an old client, how long have they worked with them?
- How many locums providers does the client need?
- Why do they need locums?

First Day Orientation–Gather before You Go!

Hospital/Office

- Address
- Phone number
- Main desk phone number

Parking

- Tag required?
- If so, where is the tag obtained?

Contacts–List as many as possible.

- Name
- Position
- Phone and extension
- Cell phone

Codes–List as many as you might need.
Notes–Make them copious!

Locums Agency Who's Who

- Agency
- Address
- Phone number
- Recruiter name
- Phone number
- Cell number
- Fax number

Credentialing assistant

- Phone number
- Cell number
- Fax number

Travel coordinator

- Phone number
- Cell number
- Fax number

Other worker bees–No one is inconsequential!

Document List–Education, Internship, Residency, Fellowships, Licenses, Certifications

College Name

- Address
- Phone number
- Years attended

- Degree obtained

Medical School Name

- Address
- Phone number
- Years attended
- Degree obtained

Internship Institution Name

- Address
- Phone number
- Years attended
- Degree obtained

Residency Institution Name

- Address
- Phone number
- Years attended
- Degree obtained

Fellowship Institution Name

- Address
- Phone number
- Years attended
- Degree obtained

Licenses–List them all!

- State
- Issued
- Expiration:

DEA

- Issued
- Expiration

Board Certification

- Issuing agency
- Date
- Recertified

ACLS/ATLS/PALS, NRP, Other(s)
NPI

References–List as many as you can. Be sure to let the people know they're references! Have their correctly spelled names, addresses, phone numbers, fax numbers, and email addresses.

Credentialing Game Plan

- Hospital
- Address
- Phone Number
- Fax Number

Credentialing contact name

- Phone number
- Fax number
- Email

Agency credentialing contact

- Phone number
- Fax number
- Email

Any documents needed/date needed
Document send date/method sent

A PDF of my checklists is available to you at my website doctorlumpkin.com. Please visit and get a copy.

CHAPTER 7

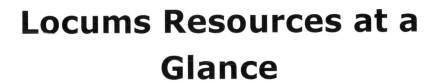

Locums Resources at a Glance

<u>NALTO</u> - National Association of Locum Tenens Organizations
<u>LocumLife</u> - An online and hard copy resource about locum tenens, its foundation and its practitioners

Traveling Tips

<u>Tripit</u> - A must-have for the frequent traveler, TripIt keeps all of your travel details in one place and provides updates and alerts when you're on the road. It's available on all platforms. It even allows you to keep all of your points from your various loyalty programs in one location.

<u>SeatGuru</u> - Aren't sure about that seat assignment you have? Look it up on SeatGuru brought to you by Tripadvisor. Not only can you find the best available seat for yourself using several

parameters, there are other useful features as well.

<u>MileIQ</u> - App for iOS or Android - Are you driving to your assignment and getting paid for your mileage? Then MileIQ offers you the easiest way to document this!

<u>Rimowa</u> – Luggage, hard-shell, highly mobile luggage.

Paperwork Partners–Work Horse Apps

<u>Shoeboxed</u> - Ever get home from a trip with a bunch of crumpled receipts and you're too tired to sort through them? Me too! I always dreaded that part of traveling, but now I have Shoeboxed. I stuff the receipts into their preaddressed mailer. When the mailer is full, I send it off. About a week later, I have a report I can review online. In no time flat, my receipts come back, pressed and neat.

<u>Evernote</u> - OK, it's not for paperwork, exactly, but if you scan anything into your tablet or computer related to work, you can store it in Evernote. The basic version is free–can't beat the cost!

<u>Scannable</u> - Available for iOS - works with Evernote (wouldn't you know?). This nifty app can scan any document you want, convert it to PDF for emailing, faxing or sending to Evernote.

<u>myCME-Bank</u> - Keep your CME/CE date current and in one place.

<u>CV updater</u> – Winway keeps your CV up-to-date.

Loyalty Programs

I know that I have mentioned this before, but it really is worth your while to join the various loyalty programs for airline, hotel and car rental. Yes, as the commercials tell you, booking rewards may not be easy, but gaining elite status will often give you perks such as earlier boarding or check-in, shorter lines, etc. If you're going to be traveling often, this can make your life that much easier.

If you do take my advice and join them, make sure that anyone doing your travel booking has those numbers available. Picking a preferred seat on a flight, another perk, is only available to elite status fliers in some cases, so keep track of those numbers and use them!

Copyright

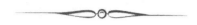

70

Made in the USA
San Bernardino, CA
16 January 2018